YOUR KNOWLEDGE HAS VALUE

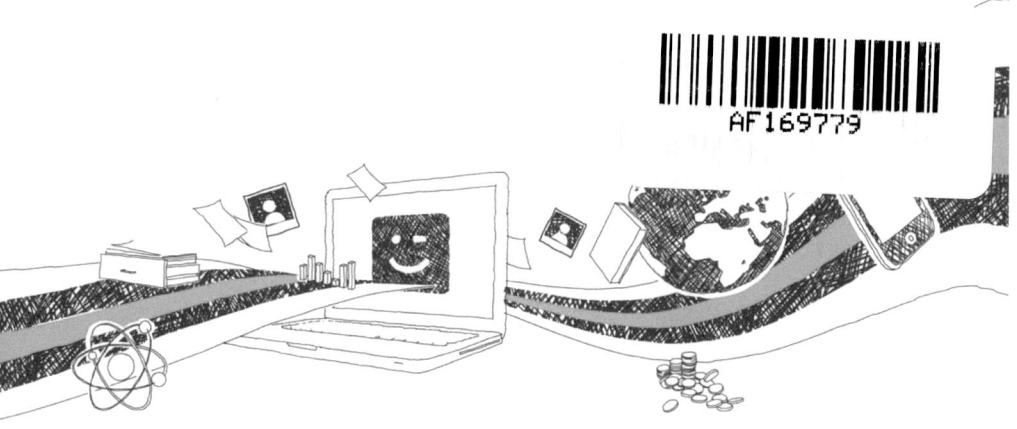

- We will publish your bachelor's and master's thesis, essays and papers

- Your own eBook and book - sold worldwide in all relevant shops

- Earn money with each sale

Upload your text at www.GRIN.com
and publish for free

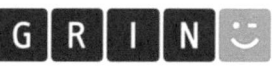

Bibliographic information published by the German National Library:

The German National Library lists this publication in the National Bibliography; detailed bibliographic data are available on the Internet at http://dnb.dnb.de .

This book is copyright material and must not be copied, reproduced, transferred, distributed, leased, licensed or publicly performed or used in any way except as specifically permitted in writing by the publishers, as allowed under the terms and conditions under which it was purchased or as strictly permitted by applicable copyright law. Any unauthorized distribution or use of this text may be a direct infringement of the author s and publisher s rights and those responsible may be liable in law accordingly.

Imprint:

Copyright © 2018 GRIN Verlag
Print and binding: Books on Demand GmbH, Norderstedt Germany
ISBN: 9783668631410

This book at GRIN:

https://www.grin.com/document/411946

Patrick Kimuyu

Understanding Type I Diabetes and the Underlying Physiological Mechanisms

GRIN Verlag

GRIN - Your knowledge has value

Since its foundation in 1998, GRIN has specialized in publishing academic texts by students, college teachers and other academics as e-book and printed book. The website www.grin.com is an ideal platform for presenting term papers, final papers, scientific essays, dissertations and specialist books.

Visit us on the internet:

http://www.grin.com/

http://www.facebook.com/grincom

http://www.twitter.com/grin_com

Understanding Type I Diabetes and the Underlying Physiological Mechanisms

Name: Patrick Kimuyu

Table of Contents

Introduction 3
Epidemiology 3
Impact of T1D on Life 3
Disease Process 4
Signs of T1D 4
Etiology of T1D 4
Genetics of T1D 5
    Cause of Beta Cells Destruction 6
    Environmental Triggers 6
    Nutritional Triggers of T1D 7
Protective Dietary Components 8
Pathophysiology of T1D 8
    Effect of T1D on Body Systems 8
Conclusion 9
References 10

Introduction

Diabetes entails a collection of metabolic disorders which are usually characterized by prolonged high sugar levels in an individual's blood. For instance, both type 1 diabetes (T1D) and type 2 diabetes (T2D) are characterized with hyperglycemia. This condition is referred as hyperglycemia, and it has been found to cause debilitating health consequences. Van Belle, Coppieters and von Herrath (2011) report reaffirm that chronic hyperglycemic conditions may lead to health complications including heart disease, blindness, kidney failure, stroke, and ketoacidosis. Ordinarily, T2D occurs due to insulin resistance in which adipose or muscle cells exhibit low response to insulin. This phenomenon is associated to old age or obesity. In contrast, T1D is caused by autoimmune destruction of pancreatic beta-cells which are responsible for the production of insulin (Ozougwu, Obimba, Belonwu & Unakalamba, 2013). Currently, diabetes presents an immense challenge to the global public health system (Kimuyu, 2018). Therefore, this discussion focuses on the key aspects of type 1 diabetes.

Epidemiology

In the US, T1D is common among children than adults. Overall, T1D has been found to occur at a prevalence rate of 1.7 per 1,000 children, primarily within 0 to 19 years age bracket (Van Belle, Coppieters & von Herrath, 2011). However, its prevalence exhibits demographic disparities. Evidence indicates that T1D affects non-Hispanic whites more than any other ethnic population (Chiang, Kirkman, Laffel & Peters, 2014).

Impact of T1D on Life

From a health lens, diabetes impacts life, adversely. Foremost, it lowers an individual's life expectancy, more or less the same as other chronic noncommunicable illnesses such as cancer, obesity and cardiovascular disease. Second, diabetes affects an individual's social life, including daily activities and career. It is also worth noting that diabetic patients experience psychosocial stress. Evidence reveals that adolescents with T1D have a high risk of developing psychosocial factors (Kakleas, Kandyla, Karayianni & Karavanaki, 2009).

Disease Process

In T1D, the disease progression is attributable to the progressive beta-cells destruction. This destruction is carried out by the body's immune system in which immune cells target Insulin-producing Islets of Langerhans, primarily the beta-cells. This autoimmune destruction leads to a decrease in the production of insulin; thus, it does not reach its normal levels in the blood. In turn, this phenomenon causes a physiological imbalance in which glucose accumulates in blood. As a result, the patient presents with T1D signs.

Signs of T1D

In practice, the onset of T1D in children is characterized by the occurrence of the principal signs. These include hunger (polyphagia), frequent urination (polyuria), accumulation of ketones in the blood (ketonemia), and excessive thirst (polydipsia). Adults present with similar signs, although it is not as acute as it is the case in children. According to clinical reports, the onset of T1D is similar to that of T2D. As such, it is relatively difficulty to diagnose T1D in adults (Chiang, Kirkman, Laffel & Peters, 2014).

Etiology of T1D

In retrospect, different epidemiological models have described the etiology of T1D. Therefore, it is apparent that that the cause of this condition has been studied extensively, in order, to understand the underlying pathophysiology of the disorder. Overall, the etiology of T1D is associated with genetic factors. However, there are environmental factors which precipitate genetic predispositions to T1D.

Genetics of T1D

Being at autoimmune disorder, T1D occurs due to changes in the genetic components in an individual's genome. Genetic mutations in the chromosomal regions involved in the production of insulin-producing genes. According to Chiang, Kirkman, Laffel and Peters (2014), there is an array of genes involved in the etiology of T1D. These include a rare monogenic forms, HLA gene, insulin gene, PTPN22 gene, IL2RA gene, and CTLA-4 gene. It is reported that T1D, hardly occurs due the mutation of a single gene, but rather a collection of genetic defects. In most cases, a single mutation combines with other autoimmune factors that are involved in the regulatory pathway to cause the disorder. For instance, genetic changes in Foxp3 transcription factor impairs the regulation of T cells; thus, leading to multiorgan autoimmunity. This phenomenon is evidenced in IPEX syndrome, as well as autoimmune polyendocrine syndrome type 1. It is estimated that 80% of children with Foxp3 mutations die early due the severity of the autoimmunity. On the other hand, genetic changes in autoimmune regulator (AIRE) have been found to cause 20% of T1D (Van Belle, Coppieters & von Herrath, 2011). Genetic changes in HLA gene have also been found to be responsible for the onset of T1D (Todd, 2010). Research indicates that more than 60% of patients with T1D posses a mutant form of HLA gene, HLA-A *0201, which increases the susceptibility for T1D. On the other hand, genetic changes in the insulin gene locus have been found to predispose individuals to T1D. Tandem repeats of VNTR type I on insulin gene locus, located on chromosome 11 impair the binding of AIRE to the promoter region, leading dysregulation. In this context, clinical studies indicate that VNTR type I is responsible for the reduced tolerance in the thymus, which is in turn caused by low transcription of insulin protein. Another essential gene involved in the development of T1D is PTPN22. This gene is concerned with the production of tyrosine phosphatase (LYP), a lymphoid protein which down regulate T cell receptor signaling. Therefore, mutations in this gene lead to the development of autoreactive T cells which are involved in the beta cells destruction (Van Belle, Coppieters & von Herrath, 2011).

Cause of Beta Cells Destruction

From a pathological perspective, the destruction of beta cells is caused by autoreactive T cells in the body. These destructive cells are known to escape from the secondary lymphoid organs, primarily the thymus where selective elimination occurs. As such, the autoreactivity of these T cells is responsible for their beta cells invasion. Therefore, it is apparent that beta cells destruction is associated to genetic factors, but not nutritional or environmental factors.

Environmental Triggers

Despite the evidence that genetic factors are responsible for the etiology of T1D, it is suggestive that environmental factors precipitate the onset of T1D. For instance, bacterial and viral infections have been found to precipitate genetic mutations into T1D. Bacteria have long been associated with physiological changes in humans, especially changes in metabolism. This phenomenon is acknowledged by Van Belle, Coppieters and von Herrath (2011) who report that microbial imbalance in the gastrointestinal tract triggers autoimmunity. It is also reported that the intestinal wall does not provide adequate protection to the immune system; thus, bacteria are able to activate the immune system. Evidence for bacterial activation of the immune system is usually provided by the presence of distorted Treg subset in the intestines of T1D patients. From a pathological perspective, the elimination of the normal intestinal microbiota exposes the immune system to activation by pathogenic bacteria.

An outstanding example of invasive bacteria that trigger the onset of T1D is the *Mycobacterium avium* subspecies paratuberculosis (MAP). This bacterium infects ruminants such as cows, and it can resist high temperatures. In humans, MAP has been found to trigger humoral responses, and its consequences include the development of mutations in SLC11A1 gene. Therefore, the expression MAP DNA in T1D patients suggests its involvement in diabetogenic responses (Dai et al., 2009).

On the other hand, some viruses have been found to trigger the onset of T1D. For instance, enteroviruses are believed to cause changes in the processing and function of the pancreatic islets. In some clinical studies, enteroviruses are isolated from the pancreatic islets, and this suggests that the infection of the beta cells by these particles results into T1D. Research indicates that enteroviruses induce the upregulation of the key proteins, primarily chemokines CXCL10. Rotaviruses are also associated with the onset of T1D. This has been reaffirmed by the presence of congenital rubella diabetes among children (Van Belle, Coppieters & von Herrath, 2011).

Nutritional Triggers of T1D

Evidence indicates that some foods or nutritional components play significant roles in the development of T1D. For instance, cow's milk is known to contain protein components that trigger autoimmunity. According to clinical reports, cross-reactivity by antibodies to beta cell surface protein (p69) and albumin occurs in infants during the early developmental stages. Therefore, feeding children with cow's milk during their early developmental stages, rather than breastfeeding predisposes them to T1D. On the other hand, wheat proteins, primarily gluten trigger T cell reactivity. According to Van Belle, Coppieters and von Herrath, (2011), gluten is linked to the onset of T1D because it initiates autoimmunity. Therefore, cow's milk and gluten-rich wheat products should be avoided in child's diet.

Protective Dietary Components

Nutrition has always been known to play significant roles in disease pathology. Despite the evidence that some dietary proteins such as gluten and albumin initiate autoimmunity in T1D, there is proof that some nutritional components are protective. For instance, vitamin D has been found to protect beta cells against autoimmune destruction. It also enhances self-tolerance; thus, preventing the development of autoreactive T cells (Van Belle, Coppieters & von Herrath, 2011).

Pathophysiology of T1D

The pathophysiology of T1D is associated to insulin deficiency which is caused by the destruction of beta cells of the pancreas. In addition, the abnormal function of the alpha cells of the pancreas potentiates the consequences of insulin deficiency. Under normal conditions, hyperglycemia reduces glucagon production by the pancreatic alpha cells. However, elevated levels of glucagon exist in T1D patients. Therefore, several biochemical mechanisms explain the principal changes responsible for tissue's response to insulin. First, insulin deficiency induces lipolysis which generates ketones and fatty acids. This explains why ketoacidosis occurs in T1D. In turn, the presence of ketones in the serum induces homeostatic responses including urination, hunger and excessive thirst (Ozougwu, Obimba, Belonwu & Unakalamba, 2013).

Effect of T1D on Body Systems

Overall, T1D affects the body negatively in different ways. It affects the excretory, endocrine, digestive, and the circulatory systems. It also affects the central nervous system. The immediate effect of T1D is the production of other endocrine hormones. For instance, insulin deficiency triggers the release of excessive glucagon levels which initiate lipid metabolism. As a result, metabolites of lipid oxidation including ketones and acids cause diabetic ketoacidosis. In addition, hormonal imbalance causes diabetic hyperglycemic hyperosmolar syndrome (Pietrangelo & Krucik, 2014).

Second, T1D affects the excretory system through the formation of kidney stones. This condition impairs the function of the kidney, primarily filtration of wastes, and it may result into irreversible kidney damage (Pietrangelo & Krucik, 2014).

Third, T1D affects the digestive system by causing gastroparesis. Hyperglycemia impairs the emptying of the stomach. This condition is known to potentiate the pathophysiology of T1D. Moreover, T1D leads to a significant disruption of the circulatory system. In most cases, T1D causes atherosclerosis, leading to the development of high blood pressure in T1D patients (Pietrangelo & Krucik, 2014).

Conclusion

Conclusively, T1D is associated with autoimmune destruction of bet cells leading to hyperglycemia. Its principal signs are polyphagia, polyuria, polydipsia, and ketonemia. Consequently, its etiology is associated with genetic and environmental triggers. Therefore, treatment of T1D focuses on glycemic control including nutritional therapy, physical activity and injection with insulin (Chiang, Kirkman, Laffel & Peters, 2014). In recommendation, future direction in the treatment of T1D should be focused on the development of vitamin D analogs.

References

Chiang, J., Kirkman, M., Laffel, L., & Peters, A. (2014). Type 1 Diabetes through the Life Span: A Position Statement of the American Diabetes Association. *Diabetes Care, 37,* 2034–2054. DOI: 10.2337/dc14-1140

Dai, Y., Marrero, I., Gros, P., Zaghouani, H., Wicker, L., & Sercarz, E. (2009). Slc11a1 Enhances the Autoimmune Diabetogenic T-Cell Response by Altering Processing and Presentation of Pancreatic Islet Antigens. *Diabetes, 58,* 156–164. DOI: 10.2337/db07-1608

Kakleas, K., Kandyla, B., Karayianni, C., & Karavanaki, K. (2009). Psychosocial Problems in Adolescents with Type 1 Diabetes Mellitus. *Diabetes & Metabolism, 35*(5), 339-350. Doi : 10.1016/j.diabet.2009.05.002

Kimuyu, P. (2018). *The State of Type 2 Diabetes and the Underlying Social, Behavioral and Psychosocial Causes.* Munich, Germany: GRIN Verlag.

Ozougwu, J. C., Obimba, K. C., Belonwu, C. D., & Unakalamba, C. B. (2013). The Pathogenesis and Pathophysiology of Type 1 and Type 2 Diabetes Mellitus. *Journal of Physiology and Pathophysiology, 4*(4), 46-57. DOI 10.5897/JPAP2013.0001

Pietrangelo, A., & Krucik, G. (2014). The Effects of Diabetes on the Body. Retrieved from http://www.healthline.com/health/diabetes/effects-on-body

Todd, J. (2010). Etiology of Type 1 Diabetes. *Immunity, 32,* 457-467. DOI 10.1016/j.immuni.2010.04.001

van Belle, T., Coppieters, K., & von Herrath, M. (2011). Type 1 Diabetes: Etiology, Immunology and Therapeutic Strategies. *Physiol Rev., 91,* 79–118. DOI:10.1152/physrev.00003.2010.

YOUR KNOWLEDGE HAS VALUE

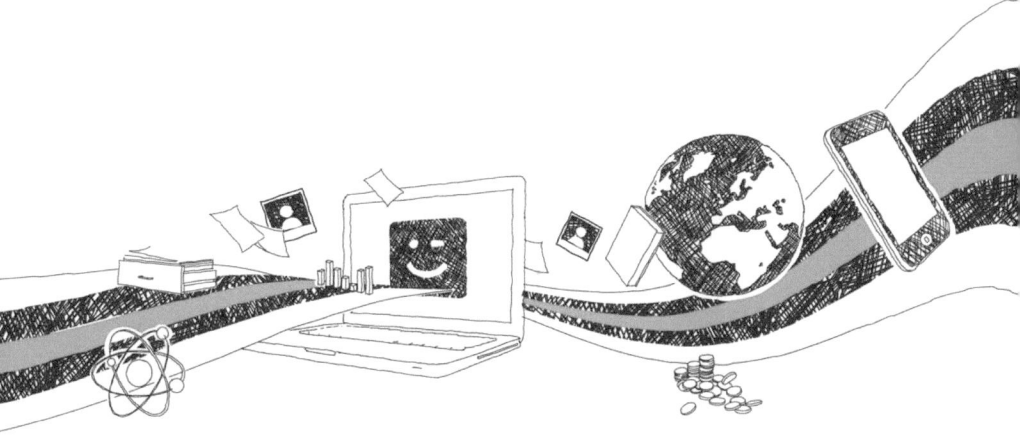

- We will publish your bachelor's and master's thesis, essays and papers

- Your own eBook and book -
  sold worldwide in all relevant shops

- Earn money with each sale

Upload your text at www.GRIN.com
and publish for free

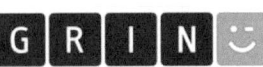